Ítalo Roger Ferreira Torres

Labour and childbirth

Ítalo Roger Ferreira Torres

Labour and childbirth

Guidelines for women and their carers

ScienciaScripts

Imprint

Any brand names and product names mentioned in this book are subject to trademark, brand or patent protection and are trademarks or registered trademarks of their respective holders. The use of brand names, product names, common names, trade names, product descriptions etc. even without a particular marking in this work is in no way to be construed to mean that such names may be regarded as unrestricted in respect of trademark and brand protection legislation and could thus be used by anyone.

Cover image: www.ingimage.com

This book is a translation from the original published under ISBN 978-613-9-65022-4.

Publisher:
Sciencia Scripts
is a trademark of
Dodo Books Indian Ocean Ltd. and OmniScriptum S.R.L publishing group

120 High Road, East Finchley, London, N2 9ED, United Kingdom
Str. Armeneasca 28/1, office 1, Chisinau MD-2012, Republic of Moldova, Europe
Printed at: see last page
ISBN: 978-620-7-84603-0

I dedicate this work to my family, who are the source of my daily inspiration and who make me seek new achievements in order to give them pride and satisfaction.

ACKNOWLEDGEMENT

I thank God in the first place for the gift of life, for faith and motivation, because without him I wouldn't have won so many victories and gained so many experiences that have added to my knowledge and given me great well-being.

To my mother Maria Auxiliadora Ferreira Torres and my father Cândido Tibúrcio Torres Neto because they have always been sources of inspiration for my achievements. Thank you for the way you brought me up, for the values and principles you showed me and for being my role models. I love you all endlessly.

The Federal University of Minas Gerais (UFMG) and the Federal University of Maranhão (UFMA), for the opportunity to take the course; the Presidente Dutra University Hospital and the Maria do Amparo Maternity Hospital for welcoming the course students to the internship field and all the teachers and preceptors involved in the course.

To my family in general, who indirectly played a part in the advice, criticism and encouragement needed for better personal and professional development.

To my friends for all their help and friendship, especially my classmates and work colleagues, Elenilda Barbosa de Jesus Dias, Luana Cristina Cardozo Souza and Marleude da Silva Xavier, you are also people who make a difference in my life and I always want to share my moments.

To my supervisor Waldeney Costa Araújo Wadie and Professor Luzinéa de Maria Pastor Santos Frias, for their guidance and suggestions in the development of this work.

Everyone played a big part in this achievement.

SUMMARY

Childbirth is considered to be a social and biological event, unique to each woman and linked to her life story, beliefs and values. Many transformations occur during pregnancy, generating anxiety and expectations in pregnant women. The presence of a carer during this period brings emotional benefits, making parturient women feel calmer and safer during the labour process. The Intervention Project aims to prepare pregnant women and their companions about labour and childbirth. The Methodology employed is Intervention Actions: Dialogue (individual and group approaches); Meetings with the Family Health Strategy Teams, with CPN Nursing Professionals. Conversation rounds with pregnant women and carers attending 21 UBS and 1 Normal Birth Centre in the municipality of Buriticupu-MA, with the aim of reflection, understanding and adherence to the Intervention Project. The first stage of the intervention was carried out between May and December 2017 with the participation of 100% of the health professionals from the UBS and CPN in the municipality of Buriticupu-MA, who approached 217 (32%) registered pregnant women. The results showed significant participation by the Municipal Coordination of Women's Health and Primary Care. Also noteworthy was the participation and contribution of the Family Health Support Centre (Núcleo de Apoio a Saúde da Familia-NASF), which boosted the project. Results: through workshops and lectures, 100% of health professionals from the UBS and the Normal Birth Centre in the municipality of Buriticupu were trained in labour and childbirth; 32% of pregnant women and their carers were involved in this project; 100% of parturients and their carers admitted to the NPC were given guidance on the institution's routine and how the process of labour and childbirth takes place.

Descriptors: Labour. Labour. Pregnant women.

SUMMARY

CHAPTER 1

INTRODUCTION

Childbirth, according to Santo and Bemi (2006), is the moment when the most intense organic and bodily changes take place, as well as the strongest emotions such as fear, pain, anxiety and joy, in a short space of time.

The pregnant woman's booklet provides various guidelines, ranging from the gestational process, bodily and emotional changes during pregnancy, labour, childbirth and the puerperium, newborn care and breastfeeding.

In the past, childbirth care was experienced as a family tradition: the presence and support of relatives and acquaintances of the woman giving birth were common practices during the birth (PINTO et al, 2003, LEÃO; BASTOS, 2001).

From the 19th century onwards, this care began to become institutionalised and medicalised due to factors including the incorporation of obstetrics into medicine and the encouragement of hospital-based medical care (LEÃO; BASTOS, 2001).

The birth process is an experience that women and their families must live through; it is historically a natural, intimate and private event that has been rethought and reformulated, mainly due to significant changes in the field of medicine. The role of the nursing professional stands out as indispensable for achieving a delivery based on humanisation, with the aim of rescuing women's autonomy (FERREIRA et al, 2017).

According to Bezerra and Cardoso (2006), preparation for childbirth is a time for health education and involves technical, educational, relational and informational procedures. The authors also stress that this time is a means of changing wrong behaviours in order to achieve better health outcomes for the pregnant woman and her family.

Health professionals should seek to maintain a helping relationship with the patient, aiming for the maternal goal and strengthening the ability of the parturient woman so that she can act effectively and satisfactorily during labour and childbirth (BEZERRA; CARDOSO, 2006). The Ministry of Health (BRASIL, 2003) ratifies this statement by defining one of the objectives of humanised care as the rescue of women as protagonists of their own condition, disengaging them from insecurity and submission to professionals in the field. Combining competent technical care with humanised care, taking into account the uniqueness, emotions and transcendent meaning of childbirth, is a necessity in the current scenario for women's care (SANTO; BERNI, 2006).

Several studies have shown that the presence of a companion with the parturient is a factor that contributes to women's satisfaction with the care they receive during labour (DOMINGUES, SANTOS; LEAL, 2004). The presence of a carer during this period brings emotional benefits, as well as helping with physical comfort measures for pain relief and providing information support for the parturient through the guidance received (LEÃO; BASTOS, 2001). For the carer to be able to offer adequate help, they need to be prepared and orientated as to their responsibilities throughout this period, remembering, however, that the carer should not be responsible for all the support because they are often also emotionally involved (EINKIN et al, 2005b). Nursing plays an important role in helping and preparing these carers to support the parturient woman, one of their aims being to make a difference to the woman's experience of pain at this time (BACHMAN, 2002).

CHAPTER 2

PROBLEMATISATION

The interest in this intervention project arose from experience and observation as an on-call nurse at the Maria de Nazaré Rodrigues Normal Birth Centre (CPNMNR), where it was observed that both the parturient and her companions are not actively involved in labour, but are only physically present at that moment, as they are still anchored in a paradigm where childbirth is centred on the professional.

The Maria de Nazaré Rodrigues CPN was inaugurated on 1st° July 2016 in the municipality of Buriticupu, the first in the state and therefore a novelty for everyone involved, as it must operate in accordance with the guidelines of the Stork Network.

Other situations were also observed at CPN Maria de Nazaré Rodrigues, such as the distancing of companions during labour, as well as the frequent request for procedures, such as the companion always asking the professional to perform the vaginal touch, the auscultation of the BCF, requesting that the parturient be assessed by the doctor and not just by nurses. In addition to situations that embarrass the woman during labour, they are not patient with the dynamics of labour and end up verbally attacking the woman, leaving her insecure. This behaviour shows not only a lack of knowledge of the hospital routine, but above all of the dynamics of labour and the humanisation of care.

Care has become depersonalised, evidenced by pre-established rules and routines, centred on the figure of health professionals, divorcing birth from a family context and from humanistic care. However, this interventionist action is undergoing a process of transition, where it aims to work with all the subjects involved during the process of pregnancy, prenatal care, childbirth and the puerperium. Therefore, labour needs to start before the parturient woman enters the NPC, incorporating actions from prenatal care in the Basic Health Units (BHUs), Because it is important that both the woman and her companion have received prior information on the subject so that they can participate more actively in pregnancy and childbirth, as well as becoming more aware of its importance and their rights, acting autonomously in their parturition process and so that when they are admitted to labour these educational measures are just a continuation so that they can minimise this anxiety, pain and stress and thus increase the degree of satisfaction of the parturient in this unique experience.

CHAPTER 3

PRESENTATION OF THE INSTITUTION

The Maria de Nazaré Rodrigues NPC opened on 1 July 2016 and is an in-hospital unit, named after the mother of the municipality's current mayor, José Gomes Rodrigues. Its team of professionals includes eleven obstetric nurses, eighteen nursing technicians and a social worker. Its structure includes an auditorium, a room for reception and risk classification (ACR), a social worker's office, five PPP suites, six shared rooms (alcon) with private bathrooms, each room containing two beds with a cot and an armchair for the accompanying person, a nursing station, a pantry and two rest rooms for the professionals. In this institution, an average of 110 babies are born every month through normal labour.

Buriticupu has a total of twenty-one Basic Health Units (UBS). Of these, eight are located in the town centre and thirteen in the countryside. All the health units have recently been refurbished and extended and have a similar physical structure, with: reception, waiting room, toilets, vaccination room, doctor's office, nurse's office, dentist's office, health agents' room, meeting room, pantry, procedure room, nebulisation, triage and observation. All of them are staffed by nurses and doctors.

CHAPTER 4

BACKGROUND

Since 1983, with the advent of the Comprehensive Women's Health Care Programme (PAISM), where teamwork and education were placed as pillars of women's health care, later with the National Comprehensive Women's Health Care Policy (PNAISM), the Humanisation of Childbirth Programme and more recently with the Stork Network strategy, a series of manuals have been produced by the Ministry of Health, which recommend that during prenatal care pregnant women receive guidance on topics such as the following: gestational process, bodily and emotional changes during pregnancy, labour, delivery and puerperium, newborn care and breastfeeding (BRASIL, 2001).

This intervention proposal is relevant for the Basic Health Units (BHU), the Birth Centre, women, families and the municipality, because health professionals at the BHU should take the opportunity to improve prenatal care, providing guidance to pregnant women and their carers on pregnancy, childbirth and the postpartum period, including: changes in the mother's body, the baby's growth and development, signs and symptoms of labour and childbirth. In this way, women will become enlightened, well-informed, safe and empowered. By participating in the process, the family will become active, expressing their feelings together with the woman, supporting her and transmitting positive thoughts.

For the professionals at the birth centre, receiving a woman who is well oriented, prepared and aware of the whole process of labour and birth will result in her having more autonomy, so that she can become the protagonist of her moment, actively participating in her birth.

As a result, the municipality also stands to gain, as the rate of normal births will increase and infant and maternal mortality rates will probably fall.

CHAPTER 5

OBJECTIVES

5.1 General

- Developing an intervention plan to prepare pregnant women and their carers about labour and childbirth.

5.2 Specific

- Prepare information material on labour and childbirth, including non-pharmacological methods of pain relief;
- Educating pregnant women and their carers about pregnancy, childbirth and post-natal care and methods of pain relief during labour;
- Sensitising health professionals on how to guide pregnant women and their carers.

CHAPTER 6

THEORETICAL FRAMEWORK

6.1 Historical evolution of labour and childbirth

Historically, the process of labour and childbirth until the 19th century was seen as a female event, accompanied and performed by midwives, who carried out this process through practical teachings that were passed down from one to another through the generations, acquiring empirical knowledge. This moment was linked to the family environment, but the presence of men was perceived as uncomfortable (SOUZA, 2015).

Also according to Souza (2015), it was from the 20th century onwards that childbirth stopped being carried out in the family and began to take place in hospitals, where scientific knowledge came to the fore.

As medicine has advanced, midwives have been sidelined and hospitals have become increasingly popular for delivering babies (MOREIRA et al, 2015). Professionals began to behave in a mechanised way, and patient care began to be carried out by countless devices, many of which replaced the physical presence of the professional. Technology is advancing and, despite its importance in care, we need to recognise its abuse (BEZERRA; CARDOSO, 2006). Based on these facts, many practices have been disregarded over time and the cultural and humanistic nature of obstetric care has been lost (LEÃO; BASTOS, 2001). The presence of a carer is an example of a practice that has been discouraged over time. In this context, experiencing the sensations of labour becomes more difficult when the woman is unaccompanied.

Currently, all over the world, fronts in favour of Obstetric Humanisation are trying to find strategies to recover labour and birth care through scientific evidence (PINTO et al, 2003). The humanisation of childbirth mainly concerns the care provided by professionals, respecting the physiological, social and cultural aspects of labour and birth, offering support to women and their families.

The presence of a family member by the parturient's side was lost as births were transferred to hospitals, but its return has been studied, since the presence of a companion stimulates a sense of well-being and comfort, and increases the parturient's satisfaction (SOUZA, 2015).

The companion in humanised childbirth is the person who provides support to the woman during the parturition process and, according to the care context, this can be represented by professionals (nurse, midwife), partner/family member or friend of the parturient (SANTOS et al,

2015).

The right to an escort was already provided for in the Prenatal and Birth Humanisation Programme, launched in 2000, before the escort law was published, and is now also reinforced in the guidelines of the Stork Network, a women's healthcare policy established in 2011 (BRUGGEMANN et al., 2014).

According to Bruggemann et al. (2014), discussions about the importance of ensuring the presence of a companion are supported by experimental studies and systematic reviews carried out in different countries from the 1980s onwards, which show the beneficial effects of support during labour.

6.2 Pregnant women's health care

Prenatal care has occupied an important place in women's health care, as it comprises a set of actions aimed at preventing, promoting, diagnosing and maintaining the health of pregnant women and newborns (GUIMARÃES, 2013).

It is important to recognise the changes that happen to women during the pregnancy cycle, even if the gestational period evolves naturally. These changes must be observed, monitored and guided by trained professionals during prenatal care. The Ministry of Health divides pregnancy into three trimesters: the first is the period when conception occurs up to 13 weeks; the second trimester is between 14 and 27 weeks; and the third trimester starts at 28 weeks (BRASIL, 2006).

In the first trimester, the main changes are nausea, vomiting, anorexia, amenorrhoea, increased heart rate, sore breasts, drowsiness, weakness, syncope, hypotension, emotional sensitivity such as the affective ambivalence of wanting or not wanting the pregnancy and fears about maternal capacity; in the second trimester, the discomforts of the first few months are not so evident; this is the moment when the pregnant woman feels the first signs of the child's vitality, in other words, the couple begins to perceive the pregnancy in a more stabilised way, both emotionally and physically, with a proportional increase in libido, which may be hindered by some taboos; in the third stage, the pregnant woman may experience cervical and lumbar pain due to the weight of the abdominal volume, the unwillingness to carry out daily activities reappears, urinary frequency increases, there is difficulty breathing, there is increased pigmentation of the vulva, the areolas, the face and the line of the lower abdomen. After 30 weeks, uterine activity increases progressively and the most intense and frequent contractions are seen in the last four weeks. During this phase, women tend to feel anxious, afraid, tired, happy, in short, they have various feelings (MANGANIELLO, 2012).

In this way, care for pregnant women and their companions should start as early as possible, guaranteeing not only care but also the establishment of a bond between the woman, her companion and the professionals, which are important for the humanisation of care (DUARTE; ANDRADE, 2008). Preparing for accompanied labour is important for identifying the right time to go to the maternity hospital. It also allows companions to feel better prepared to help during labour and birth (SOUZA and GUALDA, 2016).

The impact of this targeted care and educational activities during prenatal care also favours subsequent contact between parents and professionals in the obstetric centre and neonatal unit, as it allows both the mother and her companion to deal with difficulties and contribute to overcoming obstacles, compared to those who did not have this opportunity (GUIMARÃES, 2006). However, prenatal consultations in primary care only comply with institutional protocols that value measurements and measures, making the moment almost always routine, technical, quick and without opportunities to share knowledge and experiences (ZAMPIERI; ERDMANN, 2010).

In this way, we cannot dissociate prenatal care from educational activities at all stages of the pregnancy-puerperium cycle, since it is during prenatal care that women and their companions should be better instructed, understanding the whole evolution of pregnancy, birth and the postpartum period, since unprepared care undoubtedly becomes a complicating factor in terms of the behaviour displayed by parturients and their companions (ZAMPIERI; ERDMANN, 2010).

6.3 Guidelines for labour

6.3.1 Preparing for labour

Pregnancy, childbirth and the puerperium are a human experience with a strong positive and enriching potential for everyone who takes part. Each pregnant woman experiences her pregnancy differently. Thus, the main objective of prenatal care should be to welcome pregnant women from the outset, seeking to understand the multiple meanings of pregnancy. This is the first step towards humanised labour and birth (LAMY; MORENO, 2013).

According to Andrade (2016), a study of pregnant women investigated what they thought about childbirth and found that expectations were influenced by the experiences or stories of family and friends, most often associated with pain and suffering, especially during labour, and the most frequently mentioned expectation was the fear of not knowing the signs of childbirth, not having control over the birth, being alone and having their newborn stolen or exchanged.

It is therefore important that both the mother and her companion are informed about how labour is progressing, from the appearance of signs such as the expulsion of the mucous plug, which consists of a gelatinous, pinkish or brownish mucus with streaks of blood coming out of the vagina about 10 days or even an hour before labour; the loss of the water bag, which is the outflow of amniotic fluid from the vagina due to the rupture of the membranes surrounding the newborn, which can come out slowly or suddenly, in large quantities, is usually clear and transparent and this colour and odour should be observed and reported to the obstetrician; and regular uterine contractions, which at first are irregular and infrequent. It is also important for the parturient woman to be informed about the moment when she goes through the dilation period and culminates in the expulsive period, with the placenta coming out (SILVA, 2013).

This method involves the following stages: in the first few months of pregnancy, essential notions of the anatomy and physiology of pregnancy and childbirth should be passed on, with the aim of showing pregnant women changes in their bodies and avoiding beliefs and doubts about childbirth; in the following months, clarification should be given on: the pathophysiological mechanism of pain, as increased tension causes increased nervous system response, fear-pain; suggest the practice of muscle exercises and muscle relaxation sessions, to facilitate physical and psychological relaxation in between uterine contractions; advise on how to request the obstetrician and how to act in the process of admission to the maternity hospital; follow the stages of labour step by step; address the religious, social and psychological issues of the parturient (SILVA, 2013).

It is therefore necessary to emphasise that, in addition to providing guidance on labour, parturients should also be informed about their right to have a companion during the parturition process and the importance of this person during labour, as they represent someone with whom the pregnant woman will share her fears, who will help to minimise her anxiety and encourage her during the difficulties peculiar to labour and childbirth (SOUZA and GUALDA, 2016).

6.3.2 Care taken to relieve pain in parturient women

A number of activities can be offered to parturients and carers during antenatal care. These help parturients to manage and mitigate the pain of labour and childbirth, as they are simple methods without sophisticated equipment to use. Although not all methods are effective in relieving pain, these methods can help to reduce stress levels, such as walking, encouraging free choice of position, using the Swiss ball, breathing and relaxation exercises, bathing in the shower with warm water, massages, as well as encouraging positive feelings during labour.

Studies claim that walking can reduce the need for the dose of anaesthetic and oxytocin used and an "analgesic effect" occurs, since standing or walking can affect the perception of pain by possibly reducing traction and pressure on the roots of the lumbosacral plexus and the skeletal muscles of the pelvis during uterine contractions, by improving uterine contractility, blood flow to the fetus via the placenta is more abundant, and labour is shorter and less painful (ALMEIDA, 2015).

In addition to walking, women should also be encouraged to choose positions that make them more comfortable, as some positions promote less pain due to the change between gravity, uterine contractions, the foetus and the pelvic region. This can stimulate the progress of labour and pain relief (GOMES, FARIA E SOUZA, 2011).

In this way, Cunha (2007) reinforces the importance of nursing guidance on the use of free choice of positions, so that parturients come to understand the mechanisms of birth and can conclude that the upright position naturally favours the baby's exit due to the force of gravity.

Although the upright position was favoured in ancient times, with the opening of hospitals and maternity wards, the posture of these women during labour and childbirth began to change. At first, the lying down or reclining posture was recommended only for the moment of childbirth, but over the next three centuries, its use was extended to labour. As a result, women were admitted into labour and placed in the lithotomic position, remaining lying down throughout the process (MAMEDE; MAMEDE and DOTTO, 2007).

It is therefore important for parturient women to know about maternal posture during labour and its benefits, as it facilitates the birth process. There are two types of positions with their variations. There is the vertical position with the variations of squatting, sitting and hands-kneeling, which indicate a significant increase in the interspinous, intertubercular and coccygeal-subpubic diameters and are more suitable for physiological births, and the other position is horizontal, which are generally more suitable in cases of obstetric births and/or hypotension, which are the supine position or dorsal lithotomy and the French position or left leteral, also known as Sims (CUNHA, 2015).

Another non-pharmacological practice used for pain relief is the Swiss ball, which can be used during labour to promote more active participation by pregnant women during the parturition process (OLIVEIRA and CRUZ, 2013).

As the uterus grows, the pelvis tilts forward, accentuating the lumbosacral curvature and causing a change in the centre of gravity. This lordosis overloads the lumbar and posterior thigh muscles, generating a painful process such as postural algias (back pain) and lumbar algias (pain in the lumbar region), which are common during pregnancy and especially in the last three months, when they become more intense during labour (CUNHA, 2015).

When the parturient woman sits on the obstetric ball (Swiss ball), she has the possibility of squatting and according to Cunha (2015) this squatting position widens the pelvic angle by around 30% and facilitates expulsive efforts as the vagina widens and shortens, making it easier for the foetus to descend into the birth canal, as well as providing more comfort between and during contractions, pain relief and the physiological process of birth (D A VIM et al, 2008).

Breathing exercises during labour have the function of reducing painful sensations, improving maternal blood saturation levels of 02, providing relaxation and reducing anxiety (QUITANA et al, 2011).

Some physiological changes in the respiratory system are cited by Cunha (2015) apud Brandem (2000): Elevation of the diaphragm by up to four centimetres hindering lung expansion, replacement of the abdominal breathing pattern by thoracic breathing, increased vascularisation of the upper respiratory tract, acceleration of the respiratory rate in the last trimester, increase in the amount of air inhaled and exhaled by around 40% more, among other changes.

According to Quitana et al. (2011), it is important to emphasise that during uterine contractions, slow thoracic breathing should be prioritised, with deep and long inhalations and exhalations, in order to avoid hyperventilation. Although breathing exercises mainly reduce painful sensations during the first stage of labour. They are also effective in reducing anxiety and improving maternal oxygen saturation levels.

The aim of relaxation exercises is to allow parturients to recognise the parts of their body, highlighting the differences between relaxation and contraction, improving muscle tone and thus favouring the progress of labour (QUITANA et al, 2011). Some studies also indicate that relaxation reduces oxygen consumption, heart and respiratory rates, the concentration of lactate in arterial blood and the activity of the sympathetic nervous system (COSTA et al, 2013).

Fear and tension are the main causes of pain at the time of labour, as described by some authors during childbirth preparation courses that guide women through breathing and relaxation techniques. According to Cunha (2015), increasing women's knowledge about labour and birth, strengthening their self-confidence and sense of control, preparing a person to provide support and teaching them physical conditioning and breathing for relaxation are important measures to reduce these two factors.

Showering with warm water has increasingly been used as a method of pain relief during labour. Although few studies have proven the effectiveness of showering, it does have an influence on pain and the progress of labour, as water has beneficial and analgesic characteristics. The use of water varies greatly and can be used in various ways such as showers, baths, hydromassage and in swimming pools to carry out water births (GOMES; FARIA; SOUZA, 2011).

According to Cunha (2015) "the beneficial and analgesic properties of water have long been acclaimed, and in recent years it has aroused great interest in study in response to requests from pregnant women for this form of comfort".

In addition to analgesia, immersion in water helps to lower blood pressure, increase dilation of the cervix, relieve pain during labour, reduce trauma to the perineum and reduce oedema (GOMES; FARIA; SOUZA, 2011).

The effect of heat during bathing ends up stimulating and redistributing muscle blood flow, reducing pain and favouring muscle relaxation. According to Cunha (2015), this comfort and relaxation occurs due to the decrease in adrenaline secretion and increase in oxytocin and endorphin levels that the use of heated water promotes.

Physical touch and massage convey pain-relieving messages, depending on the way it is carried out. However, the aim of massage in labour is to enable women to relax and relieve pain, as well as reducing emotional stress and improving blood flow and tissue oxygenation. This sensory stimulation is promoted through systemic touch and tissue manipulation (GOMES; FARIA; SOUZA, 2011).

Massage can be applied to any area where the parturient reports discomfort and can also be combined with other therapies, and it is important that these massage techniques are alternated during the period of uterine contractions in order to provide relaxation (QUITANA et al, 2011), but the part of the body that most parturients usually complain of pain during labour is the lumbar region, as it is an area with great muscular tension during labour. (GOMES; FARIA; SOUZA, 2011) and according to Cunha (2015) improvements in the wellbeing of parturients were noted with circular massages with the palm of the hand in the lumbosacral region.

Despite the few studies on the movements involved in relieving pain during labour, the Ministry of Health not only encourages massages for pain relief, but also classifies this practice as demonstrably useful and should be encouraged in normal childbirth care, as it also works in the psycho-emotional aspect, because it conveys a message of interest to the recipient, of being close and wanting to help, cooperating in the interaction of the companions and the pregnant woman (CUNHA, 2015).

These approaches should be carried out during prenatal care, but many women do not have access to this guidance during pregnancy, but during admission to labour, regardless of whether the woman or her companion receives prior information on the subject. Nurses can teach or reinforce the techniques while labour is progressing, so that women receive the follow-up and support they need to minimise anxiety, pain and stress, and increase their level of satisfaction with the experience (CUNHA, 2015).

6.3.3 The pain of normal labour

Davim; Torres; Dantas, (2009) conceptualised the word pain as a sensory, emotional, degradable experience, associated with tissue damage, surrounded by painful stimuli, giving no pleasure at that moment. Childbirth, on the other hand, is characterised by the birth of the baby, i.e. the end of the pregnancy; more precisely, the literature also defines childbirth as the start of uterine contractions that produce the effacement and cervical dilation of the cervix (Almeida, 2015).

Childbirth is considered one of the critical moments for women, due to the fear and anxiety that this phase brings, as well as the physiological process of labour itself and the exogenous factors that will be acting together (TRIGOLO, 2011).

The process of pain evolution is associated with the evolution of labour, and it is mainly in the first two periods (dilation and expulsion) when parturients report the pain they feel, due to the power of the uterine contractions and the dilation of the cervix to expel the foetus (CUNHA, 2007). According to Costa et al (2006), the dilation period is divided into two phases: the latent phase, which is characterised by variable duration and irregular contractions, slow dilation, less than 1 cm/hour, and the active phase, which shows rapid dilation, equal to or greater than 1 cm/hour and regular, painful contractions. It is precisely in this phase that the greatest discomfort occurs, such as: pain in the abdominal, lumbar and pelvic regions and a sensation of fetal muscle stretching (CUNHA, 2007).

For this reason, some techniques are needed to relieve this pain. The techniques used can range from pharmacological methods such as spinal anaesthesia to non-pharmacological methods such as breathing techniques. It is often these methods that can help the parturient to relax during active labour (ALMEIDA, 2015).

Thus, nursing staff need to understand the process of labour in order to provide both parturients and their companions with an understanding of the phenomena so that they can promote physical and emotional comfort to relieve pain, as well as the anxiety and fears of this moment (CUNHA, 2007). According to the Ministry of Health (Brazil, 2003), knowledge destroys fear, avoids tension and is a strong predisposing factor for controlling pain.

5.4 The importance of the carer in this process.

In order to reduce the anxiety and fear of parturient women in labour and contribute to the humanisation of childbirth, the participation of a companion in the woman's parturition process has been encouraged. This has been ensured by law 11.108 of 2005, which regulates the presence of a companion during the entire period of labour and also guarantees that this companion must be chosen by the parturient woman (BRUGGEMANN et al, 2013).

It is believed that the experience of women who had the opportunity to have someone they chose by their side during the labour process is different from those who experienced it alone. According to PAHO (2013), during a survey of women who received continuous support during labour, they were more likely to have a spontaneous vaginal birth and less likely to receive regional analgesia, have an instrumental vaginal birth, have a caesarean section and report dissatisfaction with the birth experience, because in the hospital environment, although the woman is attended by professionals, their presence is not continuous, since the professional may be accompanying more than one woman in labour. Therefore, some countries, observing this moment, have started to promote continuous support, i.e. individual care through the support of a spouse, a relative or a person chosen by the woman, making this labour more individualised and humanised.

Therefore, humanising childbirth would mean giving women freedom of choice and providing care focused on their needs, but many are unaware of their rights to humanised childbirth, as the parturient woman not only has the right to have someone from her family present to accompany the birth, but she also has the right to receive guidance on the birth and the procedures that will be adopted, as well as freedom of movement during labour; the choice of position for the end of labour; and relaxation to relieve pain and immediate mother-baby contact immediately after birth (MOURA et al, 2007).

According to Oliveira et al (2011), the Ministry of Health recognises that the presence of a companion brings benefits and that pregnant women who have a companion during labour and the immediate puerperium are calmer and safer during the process, with a reduction in labour time and the number of caesarean sections. This humanised care for the parturient woman is important to promote a healthy labour and birth, as the health team has a defined place in childbirth care and therefore needs to recognise the potential of the companion and the benefits of their support for the woman during the parturition process, which vary according to hospital institutions (LONGO; ANDRAUS; BARBOSA, 2010).

In this context, respect for the parturient woman's wishes and rights is essential, including comfort, safety and well-being, as well as adequate pain control during labour and the presence of a companion chosen by the woman, because during pregnancy and especially during the labour and delivery process, the support obtained from the companion is important for the woman to feel more confident during this very significant and intense moment, because they usually find themselves in an unknown environment surrounded by strange people, in addition to the fear of suffering during labour, which ends up scaring the parturient woman even more. At this time, finding someone close to them who can comfort and encourage them during labour is very important (GOMES; FARIA; SOUZA, 2011).

However, it is essential that carers are included in the context of pregnancy from the outset, and that they have access to educational activities so that they can actually contribute to the parturient woman and thus contribute in a broader and more meaningful way to the woman and the moment she is experiencing, so that the carer is not only physically present, but can interact and be active in their work (MESQUITA et al., 2014).

The presence of the companion provides the emotional support that the woman needs to experience this moment, offering comfort and encouragement, which reduces feelings of loneliness, anxiety and stress levels caused by the woman's vulnerability and other factors, such as discomfort during labour, fear of what is to come, unfamiliar surroundings and contact with unknown people (MESQUITA et al, 2014). Therefore, both the professional and the carer must be able to provide information to relieve tension, meet the needs of the woman in labour and facilitate interaction between the woman, her family and the healthcare team.

In addition, Oliveira et al (2011) report that having another person with the woman also helps to reduce the risk of post-natal depression. The carer can also help the woman with basic tasks with the baby in the post-natal period, when the mother is in the rehabilitation phase.

CHAPTER 7

GOALS

- Train 100 per cent of the health professionals at the UBS and CPN in the municipality of Buriticupu through workshops or lectures, so that they become multipliers and pass on the guidelines to new pregnant women and their carers during prenatal care and childbirth;
- Involving 100% of pregnant women and their carers treated at the municipality's UBS in guidance on labour and childbirth during prenatal care;
- Educate 100% of parturient women and their companions admitted to the NPC about the institution's routine and how the labour and delivery process takes place.

CHAPTER 8

METHODOLOGY

8.1 Approach and method

We used the Intervention Project study, which is a proposal for action based on a reading of reality, considering the context. It aims to bring about change in a given organisational environment. An intervention project is made up of important elements, such as: defining priority themes; analysing the context; defining guidelines and decision-making; defining a network of tasks; and analysing the practice or result (OLIVEIRA; VIEIRA, 2014).

8.2 Intervention project site

This project was carried out in the municipality of Buriticupu-MA, which is located in the western region of the state. The municipality has an average altitude of 200 metres above sea level and geographical coordinates 4° 20'45" south latitude and 46° 24' 03" west longitude, 417 km from the capital, which can be reached via the BR 222 MA paved road. The region's predominant climate is tropical (hot and humid) with an average annual rainfall of 1,550mm, predominantly in the rainy season, from November to May. Its economy is based on agriculture and commerce. Its estimated population in 2016 was 71,227 (AGUIAR, 2015).

8.3 Target audience

Pregnant women and their carers attending the UBS in the municipality of Buriticupu - MA, family health teams, CPN nursing professionals.

8.4 Strategies and procedures

STAGE 1: SITUATIONAL DIAGNOSIS

Firstly, a diagnosis was made of the situation at the Normal Birth Centre and I observed that the pregnant women admitted had not received any guidance on labour and childbirth during prenatal care, that there were no rounds of talks to try to clear up any doubts and that they were also unaware of the right to a companion throughout labour and childbirth.

STEP 2: SEARCH FOR PARTNERS

Faced with this situation, I went in search of partnerships to improve the care provided to pregnant women from prenatal onwards.

I presented the problem to the CPN coordinator, after which I sought the support of the Primary Care and Women's Health coordinators, and then the proposal was presented to the municipal health secretary, who promptly pledged to support the project.

STEP 3: PRESENTATION

In May 2017, I met with the town's primary care nurses to make them aware of the proposed intervention and to get them to collaborate with the project, with the aim of scheduling meetings with the pregnant women registered in their units and inviting a companion of their choice. Everyone accepted the proposal and committed to helping. We discussed why pregnant women weren't given information about labour during prenatal care; the right to choose a companion during childbirth; the presence of this companion during prenatal care appointments; their visit to the place indicated for childbirth, to get to know the environment and receive guidance, etc.

According to the proposal and taking into account the proposed topics to be covered at the meetings, it was decided that the topics covered would be: signs and symptoms of labour, non-pharmacological pain relief methods, positions for labour, the law of the companion and their importance throughout the labour process. It was also agreed that the pregnant women would be divided up by trimester, i.e. first the meeting would take place with the first trimester pregnant women, then the second trimester pregnant women and finally the third trimester pregnant women, after which they would be taken to see the place indicated for labour, together with their companion.

At the time of the antenatal appointment, pregnant women were approached about taking part in the groups, and they were also approached by community health workers during home visits, who handed out invitations, which were made up individually for the pregnant woman and another for the carer, with the aim of making them feel the importance of taking part in the meetings.

During the course of the project, participants from another health programme were also invited to take part, contributing to the proposal: the NASF, made up of a psychologist, a nutritionist, a physical educator, a social worker and two physiotherapists. In July, the professionals from this programme began providing guidance at the Colégio Agrícola and Portelinha BHUs to pregnant women registered at these two health units.

In August, it was the turn of pregnant women and carers from the Centre and Caeminha units to receive guidance on labour and childbirth, which took place in two shifts due to the greater number of participants.

In August, it was agreed with the birth centre coordinators that groups of pregnant women and their companions would be taken to visit the place where the women were likely to give birth.

The normal birth centre was therefore presented to this first group from the Colégio Agrícola BHU so that they could see the facilities and receive some guidance on childbirth. Pregnant women from the Portelinha, Centro, Caeminha and Primavera health units also visited the birth centre.

In September, the project was presented to the coordinator of the normal birth centre and the professionals who work there, so that they could learn about what is being done in the municipality's UBSs with the pregnant women who will be admitted to the institution in the future.

In October, it was the turn of the pregnant women and carers registered at UBS Primavera to take part in the activity and learn about the project.

In December I met for the last time with the professionals involved in the project to present the data on the intervention and discuss the continuity of the project in the municipality.

CHAPTER 9

PRELIMINARY RESULTS

Of the twenty-one UBS in the municipality, the intervention took place in only five units (Colégio Agrícola, Portelinha, Centro, Caeminha and Primavera), all located in the municipality's headquarters.

According to SISPRENATALWEB, between 01/01/2017 and 31/12/2017, 678 pregnant women were registered in the municipality of Buriticupu, of whom 217 took part in the project. The goal was to involve 100% of registered pregnant women, but only 32% took part in the project (as shown in the graph below).

All the professionals involved in this project took part in the training workshops (100%) and all parturients and accompanying women received guidance on labour within the institution (100%).

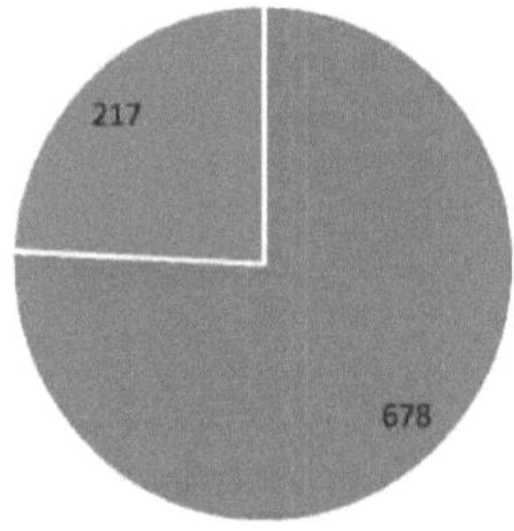

Source: SISPRENATALWEB, 2018.

The factors that made it difficult for 100 per cent of women not to adhere to guidance during pregnancy were the large number of pregnant women registered in the municipality (678), the short time available for the intervention and the little contribution of the ESF nurses in holding meetings to provide guidance to pregnant women in their areas. Even so, the project will continue.

CHAPTER 10

SCHEDULE OF ACTIVITIES

ACTIVITIES	MONTH 05/2017	MONTH 06/2017	MONTH 07/2017	MONTH 08/2017	MONTH 09/2017	MONTH 10/2017	MONTH 11/2017	MONTH 12/2017	MONTH 01/2018
Bibliographical research	▓	▓	▓	▓					
Meeting with the health professionals involved in the project	▓								
Preparation of training lectures		▓	▓						
Training for health professionals			▓						
Start of health education talks to the community			▓	▓	▓	▓			
Final analysis of the action							▓	▓	
Project presentation									▓

BUDGET

MATERIALS	QUANTITY	UNIT VALUE	TOTAL
A4 paper	02	R$ 11,00	R$ 22,00
Black ink cartridge	01	R$ 80,00	R$ 80,00
Colour ink cartridge	01	R$ 100,00	R$ 100,00
Binding	03	R$ 3,00	R$ 9,00
GRAND TOTAL			**R$ 211,00**

CHAPTER 11

FINAL CONSIDERATIONS

It is hoped that the development of this project will help to improve the quality of care provided to pregnant women and women in labour, as well as the approach to their companions so that more humanised care can be provided. Not forgetting professional enrichment, as this resource will act as a strategy for better monitoring of these pregnant women, as well as establishing a greater relationship between professionals, pregnant women and carers so that they can also take an active role during labour and childbirth.

REFERENCES

AGUIAR, I.N. **Buriticupu - its history, geography and general characteristics - 42 years of foundation and 21 years of political emancipation.** Buriticupu: Gráfica Kairós, 3ª ed, 2015.

ALMEIDA, F.M.S. **CONTROL OF PAIN IN NORMAL LABOUR:** the importance of the nurse's role. Monograph. Paulista University. Graduation in Nursing, São José dos Campos, 2015. Available at: < http://www.ebah.com.br/content/ABAAAhFz8AC/tcc-dor-no-trabalho-parto-parto-normal- importancia-atuacao-enfermeiro >. Accessed on: 10 October 2017.

ANDRADE, I. S. **Validation of an educational video for the knowledge, attitude and practice of pregnant women in preparation for active labour,** 2016. 85fi: il. Tese (doutorado) - Universidade Federal do Ceará; Centro; Faculdade de Farmácia, Odontologia e Enfermagem; Departamento de Enfermagem; Programa de Pós-Graduação em Enfermagem; Doutorado em Enfermagem, Fortaleza, 2016.

BACHMAN, J.A. Discomfort management. In: LOWDERMILK, D.L; PERY. S.E; BOBAK, LM. **Maternal nursing care.** 5ª ed. Porto Alegre: Artmed, 2002, p. 314-35.

BEZERRA, M.G.A; CARDOSO, M.V.L.M.L. **Factores culturais que interferem nas experiencias das mulheres durante o trabalho de parto e parto.** Revista Latino-americana, v. 14, n. 3, p. 414-421, mai/jun. 2006.

BRANDEM, P.S. Physiological and psychosocial changes in normal pregnancy. In:. **Enfermagem Materno Infantil.** 2ª ed. Rio de Janeiro/RJ: Reichman & Affonso, 2000.

BRAZIL. Ministry of Health. Secretariat for Health Policy. Health Technical Area Women. **Childbirth, abortion and the puerperium: humanised care for women** / Ministry of Health, Secretariat for Health Policies, Women's Technical Area. - Brasília: Ministry of Health, 2001.

BRAZIL. Ministry of Health. **Childbirth, abortion and the puerperium:** humanised health care. Brasília-DF: Ministry of Health, 2003, p. 199.

BRAZIL. Ministry of Health. Maternal and Child Health Coordination. Comprehensive Women's

Health Care Programme. **Prenatal Care: Technical Manual.** 3. Ed. Brasília, 2006.

BRUGGEMANN, O. M. et al. **The inclusion of birth companions in public health services in Santa Catarina, Brazil.** Rev. Esc. Anna Nery, 2013, Jul/Sep; 17 (3): 432-438. Disponível em: http://www.scielo.br/pdf/ean/vl7n3/1414-8145-ean-17-03-0432.pdf. Accessed on: 18 November 2016.

BRUGGEMANN, O. M. et al. **Reasons why health services do not allow birth companions:** nurses' discourses. Florianópolis, 2014. Available at:<http://www.scielo.br/scielo.php?pid=S010407072014000 200270&script=sci_arttext&tlng=en>. Accessed on: 22 November 2016.

COSTA, S.H.M et al. **Assistance in labour.** Routines in obstetrics. 5º Ed. Porto Alegre- RS: Armed, 2006, p. 231-246.

COSTA, M.M.N et al. **USE OF NON-PHARMACOLOGICAL METHODS TO ALLEVIATE PAIN DURING NORMAL LABOUR:** integrative review. Revista de Enfermagem UFPE, 2013, v.7, pag. 4161-4170. Available at:
<http://www.revista.ufpe.br/revistaenfermagem/index.php/revista/article/viewFile/2582/pdf_2 608>. Accessed on 30 October 2017.

CUNHA, M.L.K. **Orientations for carers of women in labour:** a proposal for health education. 2007. 42 f. Final Course Work (Bachelor's Degree in Nursing).
Federal University of Rio Grande do Sul, Porto Alegre, 2007. Available at:
<http://www.lume.ufrgs.br/bitstream/handle/10183/107817/000605587.pdf?sequence= 1 >. Accessed on: 18 November 2016.

DA VIM, R. M. B. et al. **Showering as a non-pharmacological strategy for pain relief in parturients.** Revista Eletrónica Enfermagem, 2008;10(3):600-9.

DA VIM, R.M.B; TORRES, G.V; DANTAS, J, C. **EFETIVIDADE DE ESTRATÉGIAS NÃO FARMACOLÓGICAS NO ALÍVIO DA DOR DE PARTURIENTES NO LABOR.** Revista da Escola de Enfermagem da USP, 2009, Jun, v.43, n° 2. Available at:
<http://www.scielo.br/scielo.php?script=sci_arttext&pid=S0080- 62342009000200025 >. Accessed on: 10 November 2017.

DOMINGUES, R.M.S.M; SANTOS, E.M; LEAL, M.C. **Aspectos da satisfação das mulheres com a assistência ao parto: contribuição para a debate.** Cadernos de Saúde Pública, Rio de Janeiro, v. 20 Suppl. 1, p. S52-S62, 2004.

DUARTE, S. J. H.; ANDRADE, S. M. O. **The meaning of prenatal care for pregnant women:** an experience in the municipality of Campo Grande, Brazil. Rev. Saúde Soc., v.17, n° 2, pag. 132-139, Apr./Jun. 2008.

. Social and professional support in childbirth. In: ENKIM, M. et al. **Guia para atenção efetiva na gravidez e no parto.** 3ª ed. Rio de Janeiro/RJ: Guanabara Koogan, 2005b, p. 133- 136.

FERREIRA, L.M.S et al. **Nursing care during labour and childbirth: women's perception. Revista Cubana de Enfermería,** vol. 33, n° 02 (2017). Available at:
http://revenfermeria.sld.cu/index.php/enf/article/view/1102/263. Accessed on: 15 December 2017.

GOMES, A.S; FARIA, J.; SOUZA, R. **HOME BIRTH: THE SEARCH FOR A HUMANISED BIRTH IN THE PERCEPTION OF A GROUP OF WOMEN.** Monograph. Faculdade Estácio de Sá de Santa Caratina, Nursing Course, São José, 2011. Available at: < http://www.equipehanami.com.br >. Accessed on: 10 October 2017.

GUIMARÃES, G. P. **The formation of parent/preterm and/or low birth weight newborn attachment in the Kangaroo Mother Method:** a nursing contribution. 2006. Dissertation

(Master's Degree in Nursing) - Postgraduate Programme in Nursing, Federal University of Santa Catarina, Florianópolis, 2006.

GUIMARÃES, G. P. **Health education as a dialogical space for the experience of high-risk pregnancy,** Florianópolis, SC, 2013. 225 p.

LAMY, G.O; MORENO, B.S. **Prenatal care and preparation for childbirth.** Revista Omnia Saúde, 2013,   v.10,   n.2, p. 19-35. Available at: < http://www.fai.com.br/portal/ojs/index.php/omniasaude/article/viewFile/456/pdf>. Accessed on: 10 December 2017.

LEÃO, M.R.C; BASTOS, M.A.R. **Doulas supporting women during labour: experiences at Sofia Feldman Hospital.** Revista Latino-americana de Enfermagem, v. 9, n. 3, p. 90-94, mai. 2001.

LONGO, C.S.M; ANDRAUS, L.M.S; BARBOSA, M.A. **PARTICIPAÇÃO DO ACOMPANHANTE NA HUMANIZAÇÃO DO PARTO E SUA RELAÇÃO COM A EQUIPE DE SAÚDE.** Revista Eletrónica de Enfermagem, 2010, v. 12, n° 2, pag. 386-391. Available at: <https://www.fen.ufg.br/fen_revista/vl2/n2/pdf/vl2n2a25.pdf>. Accessed on: 20 October 2017.

MANGANIELLO, A. **Prulho de pai: primilha** educativa para a promoção do envolvimento paterno na gravidez - Thesis (Doctorate)- Escola de Enfermagem da Universidade de São Paulo, São Paulo, 2012, 206p.

MAMEDE, F.V; MAMEDE, M.V; DOTTO, L.M.G. **REFLEXÕES SOBRE DEAMBULAÇÃO E POSIÇÃO MATERNA NO TRABALHO DE PARTO E PARTO.** Revista de Enfermagem, 2007, 11(2): 331-6. Available at: < http://www.scielo.br/pdfrean/vlln2/vlln2a23>. Accessed on: 10 October 2017.

MESQUITA, N. S et al. **THE CONTRIBUTION OF THE ASSISTANT TO THE HUMANISATION OF PARTURITION AND BIRTH:** perceptions of puerperal women. Rev. Esc Anna Nery, 2014, v. 18, n° 2, pag. 262-269. Disponível em: http://www.scielo.br/pdfrean/vl8n2/1414-8145-ean-18-02-0262.pdf. Accessed on: 20 October 2017.

MOREIRA, A. P. A. et al. **Paternal preparation to be companions in labour.** Rev. Enfermagem Obstétrica, Rio de Janeiro, 2015, Jan/Apr; 2 (1): 3-8. Available at: http://www.enfo.com.br/ojs/index.php/EnfObst/article/view/18. Accessed on: 21 November 2016.

MOURA, F. M. J. S. P. et al. **Humanisation and nursing care in normal childbirth.** Revista Brasileira de Enfermagem, Brasília, DF, v. 60, n. 4, p. 452-455, 2007.

SILVA, E.A.T. **Pregnancy and preparation for childbirth: an intervention programme.**

Revista O Mundo da Saúde, São Paulo, 2013, n37, v2, pag 208-215.

OLIVEIRA, A.S.S.O et al. **THE ACCOMPANIER IN THE MOMENT OF LABOUR AND BIRTH PERCEPTION OF PREGNANT WOMEN.** Rev. Cogitare Enfermagem, 2011, Apr/Jun; v.16, n° 2, pag. 247-253. Available at: < >. Accessed on: 13 November 2017.

OLIVEIRA, A. E. F. et al. **Manual for the organisation of course completion work.** São Luís: EDUFMA, 1ª ed, 2013.

OLIVEIRA^L.M.N; CRUZ, A.G.C. A **UTILIZAÇÃO DA BOLA SUÍÇA NA PROMOÇÃO DO PARTO HUMANIZADO.** Revista Brasileira de Ciência da Saúde, 2013, v.18, n° 2, pag. 175-180. Available at <http://periodicos.ufpb.br>. Accessed on: 15 October 2017.

OLIVEIRA, A.R.F; VIEIRA, T.F. **Processo de investigação científica** e os tipos de Universidade Federal do Maranhão. UNA-SUS/UFMA knowledge - São Luís, 2014.

PAN-AMERICAN HEALTH ORGANISATION. Basque Government, Central Publishing Service. **Clinical practice guide on normal childbirth care.** Restricted version. Brasilia, DF: PAHO, 2013.

PINTO, C.M.S. et al. **The labour companion: activities developed and evaluation of the experience.** Revista Mineira de Enfermagem, Minas Gerais, v. 7, n. 1, p. 41-47, jan/jul, 2003.

QUITANA, S.M et al. **NON-PHARMACOLOGICAL RESOURCES IN LABOUR:** care protocol. FEMINA, 2011, Jan. v.39; n° 1.

SANTOS, A. L. S. et al. **The companion in labour from the perspective of the puerperal woman.** Rev. Enferm. UFSM, 2015, Jun/Set; 5 (3): 531-540. Available at: https://periodicos.ufsm.br/index.php/reufsm/article/view/17337. Accessed on: 18 November 2016.

SANTO, L.C.E; BERNI, N.I.O. Nursing in Obstetrics. In: Freitas et al. **Routines in Obstetrics.** 5ª ed. Porto Alegre: Artmed, 2006.

SOUZA, M.A.R. **Parturient companion's experience of the labour and delivery process.** Dissertation (Master's in Nursing). Postgraduate programme in nursing, Federal University of Paraná, Curitiba, 2015. Available at: http://acervodigital.ufpr.br/bitstream/handle/1884/41367/R%20%20D%20%20MARLI%20A PARECIDA%20ROCHA%20DE%20SOUZA.pdf?sequence=2&isAllowed=y. Accessed on: 21 November 2016.

TRIGOLO, C.M. **CASA DE PARTO: a** reference point for overcoming the fear and perspectives of pregnant women. Monograph. Municipal Institute of Higher Education of Assis/ IMESA. Educational Foundation of the Municipality of Assis/ FEMA. Assis, 2011. Available at: < >. Accessed on: 10 October 2017.

SOUZA, S.R.R.K; GUALDA, D.M.R. **A EXPERIÊNCIA DA MULHER E DE SEU ACOMPANHANTE NO PARTO EM UMA MATERNIDADE.** Texto Contexto Enferm, 2016; V. 25, N.1

ZAMPIERI M.F.M; ERDMANN A.L. **Humanised prenatal care:** a look beyond divergences and convergences. Rev. Bras. Saúde Matem. Infant., Recife, v. 10, n° 3,

pag. 359-367. jul. / sep., 2010. Available at:
<http://www.scielo.br/pdf7rbsmi/vl0n3/vl0n3a09.pdf>. Accessed on: 15 December 2017.

APENDICES

APPENDIX A - Meeting with primary care nurses about the intervention project

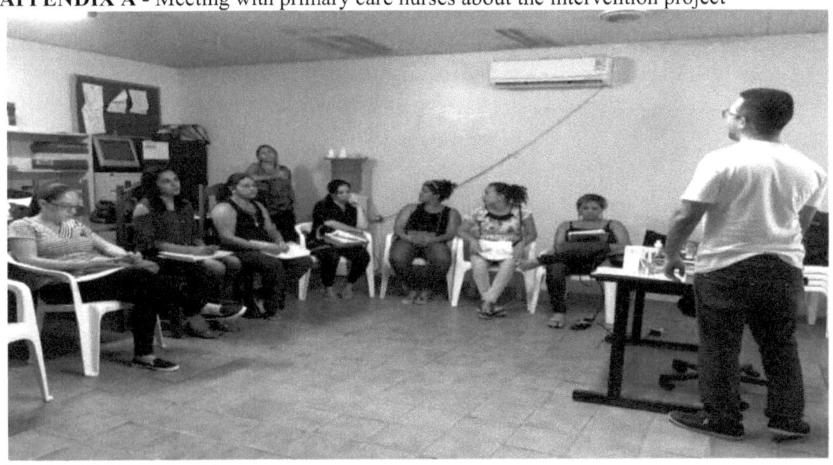

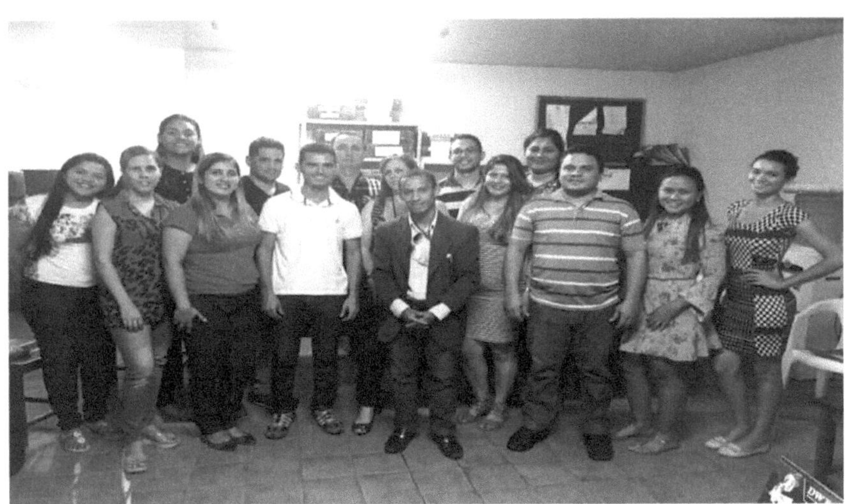

APPENDIX B - Presentation of the intervention project to CPN professionals

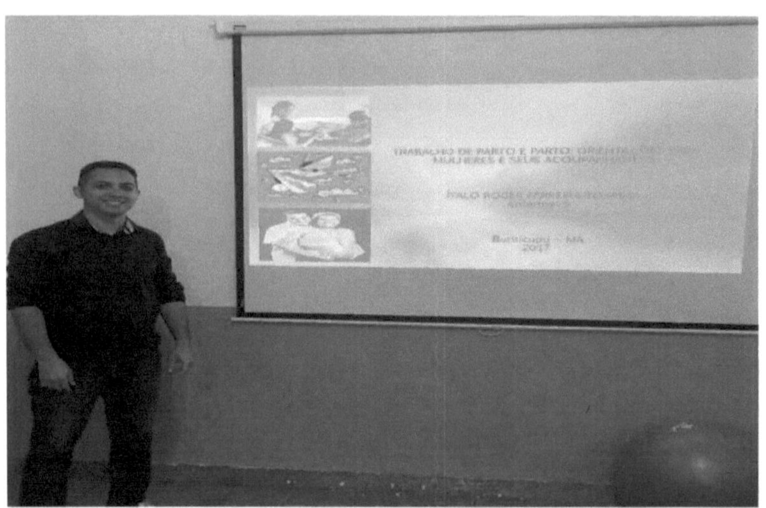

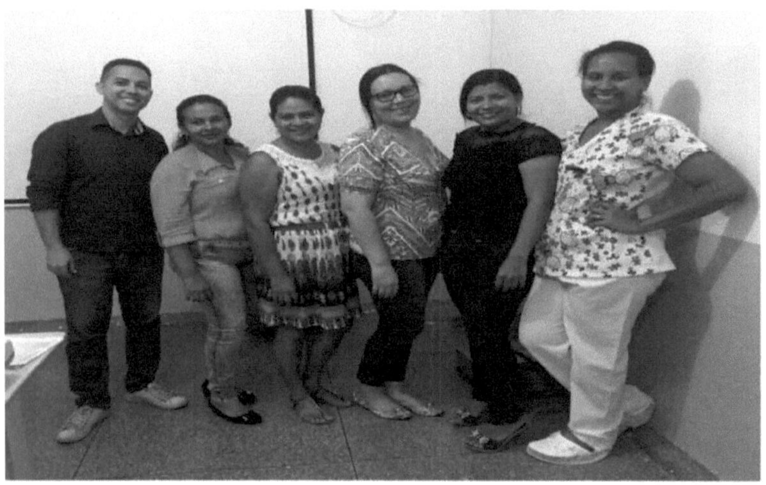

APPENDIX C - Term of Commitment signed by municipal managers

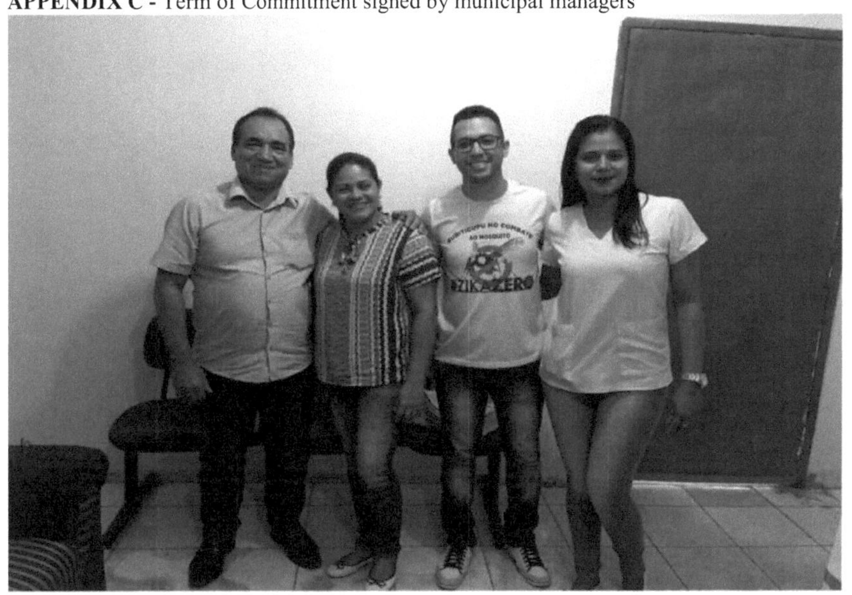

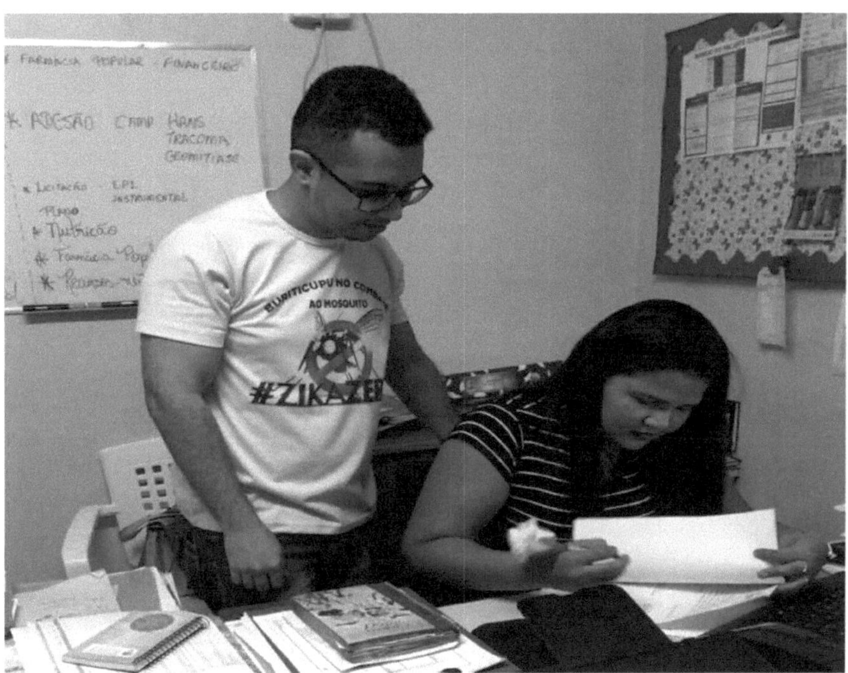

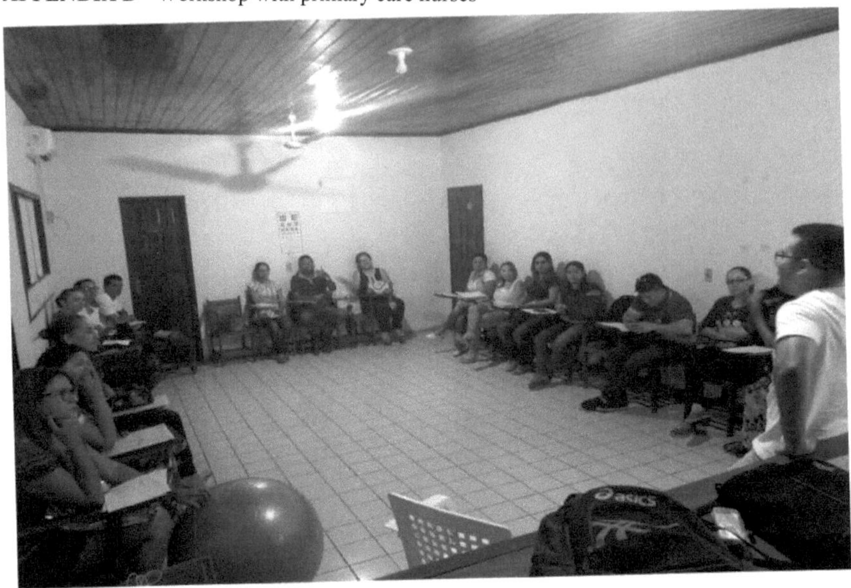

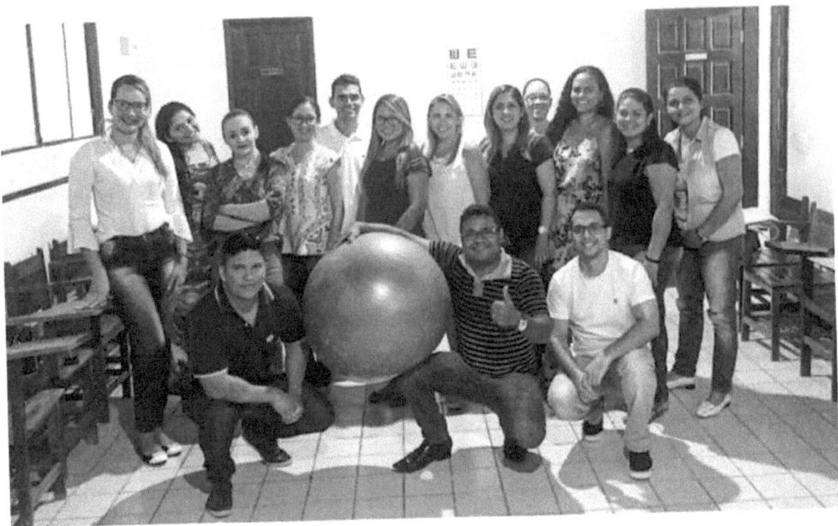

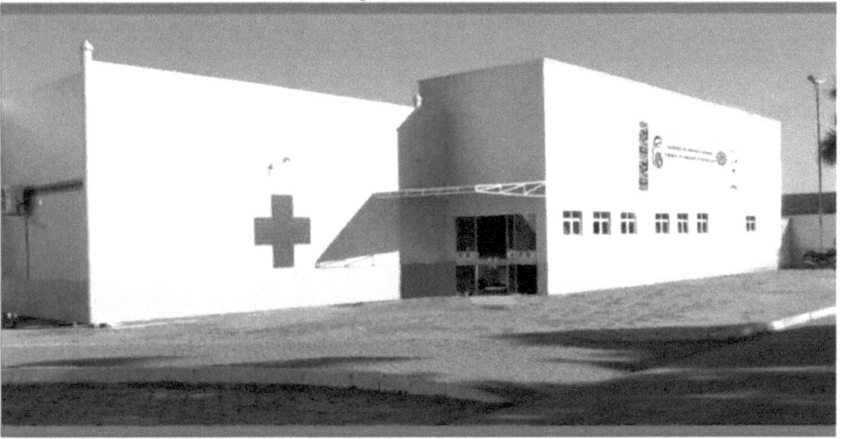

APPENDIX F - Consent form signed by the managers of the municipality of Buriticupu

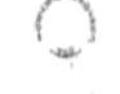

PREFEITURA MUNICIPAL DE BURITICUPU - MA
SECRETARIA MUNICIPAL DE SAÚDE
RUA SANTA MARIA, S/Nº, TERRA BELA
CNPJ: 12.036.458/0001-80

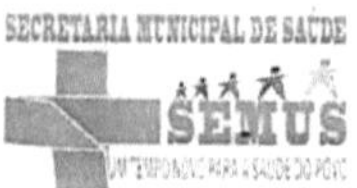

TERMO DE ANUÊNCIA

Declaramos para os devidos fins que estamos de acordo com a execução do projeto de intervenção intitulado "Trabalho de parto e parto: orientações para mulheres e seus acompanhantes", do aluno **Ítalo Roger Ferreira Torres** do Curso de Especialização em Enfermagem Obstétrica – Rede Cegonha (UFMA/UFMG). A orientação do projeto é de responsabilidade do (a) Prof (a). Ma. **Waldeney Costa Araújo Wadie,** o qual terá o apoio desta Instituição.

Buriticupu, 04 de dezembro de 2017.

____
Elias Rocha de Sousa
Secretário Municipal de Saúde

____
Edmelry Ferreira da Silva
Coordenadora da Atenção Básica

____
Acenate Fernandes
Coordenadora do Centro de Parto Normal
Maria de Nazaré Rodrigues

APPENDIX G - Frequency of professionals who took part in the Workshop on the Intervention Project

 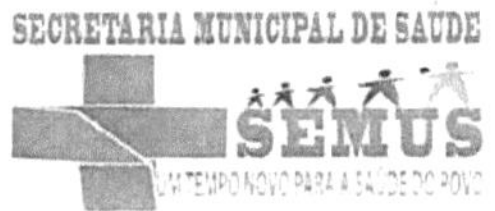

PARTICIPANTES DA OFICINA SOBRE O PI TRABALHO DE PARTO E PARTO:

ORIENTAÇÕES PARA MULHERES E ACOMPANHANTES

DATA: 14/12/2017

NOME	LOCAL DE TRABALHO	TELEFONE
Juliana Lima Gomes	UBS Vila Braias	(98) 98102 1202
Raphael Jaens Lasmirs	UBS Saude T. Bels	(98) 98461 7260
Erica Almeida Nicacio	UBS Vila Primo	(99) 98207-6065
Edna Lima Ferreira	ESF. Buritizinho	(98) 98400-6389
Marcia Maria de Sousa Lima	UBS Rubenita Macedo	(98) 98770 1611
Evangelista Fonseca da Silva	USF VILA UNIÃO / C. FARIAS	(98) 98108 4574
Franciele Santos Bahia	USF Trilha 410	(98) 98487-8955
Carla Mirelle Franco Leite	USF Rubenita Macedo	(98) 99982 6898
Solange Tavares Cruz	UBS: III VICINAL	(98) 98132 1450
Mayara S. dos Santos	II - Núcleo	(99) 98194-6441
Kelly Cristine de Souza	UBS: Dedisto Flor	(98) 99203 8020
Ketey Angela Barbosa de Oliveira	UBS Brejinho	(99) 98140 0315
Marcia Lopes dos Santos	UBS. S. Francisco	(98) 98714 2130
Mércia Mayara Espanol	U.B.S. Primavera	(99) 9843-1003
Elenilso B. J. Dias.	U.B.S L. Agrícola	(98) 9833-10 80.
Francisca Ribeiro Fidelis	UBS V. Primavera	(98) 98731-2817
Lucrécia Sousa de Lima	U.B.S VILA DAVI	(98) 98703 9502

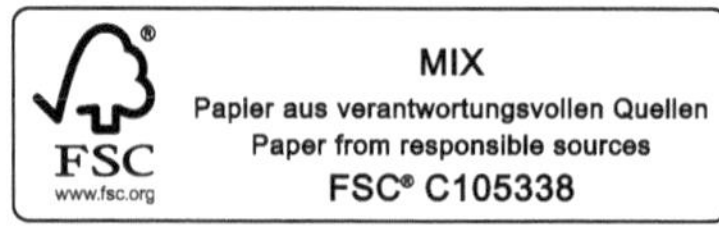

Printed by Books on Demand GmbH, Norderstedt / Germany